CHAIR PILATES FOR BEGINNERS

The complete 28 days body sculpting challenge to strengthen your muscles, tone your abs, glutes and improve your balance posture with step-by-step illustrated full body exercises.

ROBERT S MARLOW

SCAN TO GET MORE BOOKS BY THIS AUTHOR

TABLE OF CONTENT

ENJOY, ENDURE AND PROGRESS NOW!!!

INTRODUCTION

In the heart of a bustling city, where the rhythm of life never seemed to slow, lived a woman named Lily. Her days were a whirlwind of meetings, deadlines, and endless tasks. The concept of a fitness routine felt like an elusive dream, slipping through her fingers amid the demands of her busy schedule. Until one day, fate intervened in the form of a book.

Nestled between rows of neatly stacked volumes in a local bookstore, a title caught Lily's eye "Chair Pilates Strengthen Your Body, Transform Your Life." The words seemed to shimmer with possibility. With curiosity piqued, she pulled the book from the shelf, its pages promising a way to unlock vitality and wellness, all from the comfort of a chair.

As she turned the pages, Lily's skepticism transformed into intrigue. Chair Pilates, a series of exercises designed to harness the power of a simple chair, offered a solution tailored to her fast-paced life. With each description of an exercise and the accompanying illustrations, Lily could almost feel the energy and focus that Chair Pilates could bring to her routine.

Determined to break free from the monotony of her sedentary habits, Lily embraced the challenge. She cleared a space in her living room, her favorite armchair taking center stage. The book became her guide, and the chair her newfound workout companion.

The first session left her surprised. The seemingly uncomplicated movements engaged muscles she had long forgotten. The stretches brought a sense of release, and the controlled motions felt oddly liberating. What started as an experiment gradually evolved into a daily ritual.

Weeks turned into months, and Lily's transformation was undeniable. The chronic tension that once resided in her shoulders began to dissipate. Her posture, once a casualty of endless hours at a desk, now exuded confidence. And the fatigue that used to linger was replaced by a sustained sense of vitality.

Lily's journey with Chair Pilates extended beyond the physical. As she breathed through each movement, she found a space for mindfulness, a sanctuary of calm amid the chaos. The chair, once an ordinary piece of furniture, had become a catalyst for her well-being.

Her friends began to notice the changes, the vibrancy that seemed to emanate from within. Intrigued, they inquired about her secret. With a smile, Lily shared her newfound passion and the book that had set her on this path of transformation.

Soon, her living room echoed with laughter and camaraderie as friends gathered around chairs, mirroring the exercises

Lily had adopted. The chair, it seemed, had woven a thread of wellness through the lives of those she held dear.

Lily's journey was a testament to the profound impact of a single decision. Amid the demands of modern life, she had discovered a way to prioritize herself, to embrace vitality on her own terms. And as her story spread, the chair became more than an object—it became a symbol of empowerment, a reminder that even amidst the busiest of days, there's always a seat waiting for wellness.

CHAIR PILATES DESCRIPTION

Understanding chair Pilates

Chair Pilates is a form of exercise that adapts traditional Pilates movements to be performed using a chair as a prop. This modification makes Pilates accessible to a wider range of individuals, including those with limited mobility or balance issues. Chair Pilates can help improve strength, flexibility, posture, and overall body awareness.

Types of Chair Pilates

There are various types of chair Pilates exercises that target different muscle groups and areas of the body. Some common types include

1. Upper Body Chair Pilates Focusing on the arms, shoulders, and upper back.

2. Lower Body Chair Pilates Concentrating on the legs, hips, and lower back.

3. Core Chair Pilates Emphasizing the abdominal muscles and the muscles supporting the spine.

4. Full-Body Chair Pilates Integrating exercises that engage both upper and lower body muscles.

40 Pilates Exercises using a chair for beginners, along with step-by-step instructions.

(Tip: Ensure you have a good and standard chair to perform these exercises.)

1. Seated Arm Circles
- Sit tall on the edge of the chair.
- Keep your arms at shoulder height out to the sides
- Circle your arms forward and then backward, engaging your shoulder muscles.

2. Leg Lifts
- Sit upright, hands on the chair for balance.
- Keep one leg parallel to the ground while you extend it straight out in front of you.
- Lower the leg back down and switch to the other leg.

3. Seated Spine Twist
- Sit tall, cross your arms over your chest.
- Twist your torso to the right, using the chair's back for support.
- Return to the center and repeat on the left side.

4. Seated Cat-Cow Stretch
- Sit forward on the chair, hands on your knees.
- Arch your back (cow) and then round it (cat), coordinating with your breath.

5. Single Leg Circle
- Sit on the chair's edge, hands beside you for support.
- Lift one leg and make small circles in the air.
- Reverse the direction of the circles.

6. Seated Forward Bend
- Sit tall and hinge at your hips, reaching towards your feet.
- Keep your spine lengthened and avoid rounding your back.

7. Seated Side Stretch
- Sit sideways on the chair, one hand holding the backrest.
- Reach the other arm over your head, creating a stretch along your side.
- Switch sides.

8. Arm Raises
- Sit tall, holding the sides of the chair.
- Lift both arms overhead, engaging your core.
- Lower your arms back down.

9. Hip Opener
- Sit on the chair, ankle of one leg resting on the opposite knee.
- Gently press down on the lifted knee to open the hip.
- Switch legs.

10. Seated Chest Opener
- Sit tall, clasp your hands behind your back.
- Squeeze your shoulder blades together as you lift your arms slightly.

11. Leg Extensions
- Sit upright, hands resting on the chair's seat.
- Extend one leg straight out and hold briefly before lowering.
- Alternate legs.

12. Seated Roll Up
- Sit forward on the chair, hands resting on your thighs.
- Slowly round your spine, tucking your chin to your chest.
- One vertebra at a time, roll back up.

13. Knee Lifts
- Sit tall, grip the sides of the chair.
- Lift both knees towards your chest, engaging your core.
- Lower your feet back down.

14. Seated Figure Four Stretch
- Sit tall, ankle of one leg on the opposite knee.
- Gently press down on the lifted knee, feeling a stretch in your hip.
- Switch sides.

15. Side Leg Lifts
- Sit sideways on the chair, one hand on the backrest.
- Lift the top leg sideways while keeping it straight.
- Retract the leg and change sides.

16. Arm Pulls
- Sit upright, hold the chair's backrest with both hands.
- Pull your shoulder blades back as you squeeze your elbows behind you.

17. Seated Bicycle
- Sit tall, hands behind your head.
- Lift one knee towards your chest as you twist to bring the opposite elbow towards it.
- Alternate sides in a pedaling motion.

18. Seated Twist with Leg Extension
- Sit forward, hold the chair's sides.
- Lift one leg and twist your torso toward that leg.
- Twist while extending the raised leg straight out.

19. Seated Side Leg Circles
- Sit sideways on the chair, one hand on the backrest.
- Lift the top leg and make small circles in the air.
- Reverse the direction of the circles and switch sides.

20. Shoulder Shrugs
- Sit tall, arms relaxed by your sides.
- Lift your shoulders towards your ears, then release them down.

21. Seated Lateral Flexion
- Sit on the chair's edge, one hand on the seat.
- Reach the opposite arm overhead and lean to the side.
- Switch sides.

22. Seated Arm Pushes
- Sit tall, hands on the chair's armrests.
- Press your hands down, engaging your triceps, then release.

23. Leg Crosses
- Sit forward, hands resting on your thighs.
- Gently push down on the crossed knee while crossing one ankle over the other.
- Switch legs.

24. Seated Torso Circles
- Sit tall, hands on your hips.
- Circle your torso in one direction, then switch to the other direction.

25. Seated Side Leg Raises
- Sit on the chair, hands resting on the chair's seat.
- Lift one leg straight out to the side, engaging your outer hip.
- Retract the leg and change sides.

26. Arm Reaches with Rotation
- Sit tall, hands clasped in front of you.
- Reach your arms forward, then rotate your torso to one side.
- Return to the center and switch sides.

27. Seated Hamstring Stretch
- Sit tall, one leg extended straight out.
- Hinge at the hips and reach toward your extended foot.

28. Seated Hip Flexor Stretch
- Sit tall, one ankle resting on the opposite knee.
- Gently press down on the lifted knee, feeling a stretch in the hip.

29. Seated Backbend
- Sit forward, place your hands on the chair's backrest.
- Arch your spine gently, looking upwards.

30. Seated Side Leg Extensions
- Sit tall, hands on the chair's armrests.
- Lift one leg straight out to the side, engaging your outer hip.
- Retract the leg and change sides.

31. Arm Circles
- Sit tall, arms extended to the sides.
- Circle your arms forward, then backward, focusing on your shoulder muscles.

32. Seated Leg Cross Twists
- Cross one leg over the other while sitting tall
- Feel a stretch as you turn your body toward the crossed leg..
- Switch the cross of your legs and twist to the other side.

33. Seated Abdominal Twist
- Sit tall, hands behind your head.
- Twist your upper body from side to side, engaging your obliques.

34. Seated Inner Thigh Stretch
- Sit forward, feet together, knees out to the sides.
- Feel the stretch in your inner thighs as you gently press down on your knees.

35. Seated Arm Lifts
- Sit tall, hands resting on your lap.
- Lift your arms overhead, engaging your shoulders, and then lower them down.

36. Seated Neck Stretches
- Sit tall, gently tilt your head to one side, feeling a stretch in your neck.
 - Repeat on the other side and then gently forward and backward.

37. Seated Hip Circles
- Sit tall, hands on your hips
- Circle your hips in one direction, then switch to the other direction.

38. Seated Wrist and Forearm Stretches
- Sit tall, extend one arm in front of you.
- Your wrist and forearm may be stretched by gently pulling back on your fingers.
- Repeat with the other arm.

39. Seated Ankle Rolls
- Sit tall, extend one leg straight out.
- Rotate your ankle in circles, then switch to the other ankle.

40. Seated Breathing and Relaxation
- Sit comfortably, close your eyes.
- Fill your lungs with air as you inhale deeply with your nose and gently let it out through your mouth.
- Focus on your breath, allowing your body to relax.

Remember to listen to your body, and if any exercise causes discomfort or pain, stop immediately. It's essential to start slowly and gradually increase intensity as your body becomes more accustomed to the exercises. Always maintain proper form and alignment for the best results and to prevent injury.

20 motivational quotes specifically tailored for beginners in Chair Pilates

1. "Every small step you take in your Chair Pilates journey is a giant leap toward a healthier and stronger you."

2. "Beginnings are the seeds of transformation; embrace your Chair Pilates journey with enthusiasm."

3. "In the world of Chair Pilates, every beginner is a potential powerhouse of progress."

4. "With elegance, begin your Chair Pilates routine, and watch as your strength grows

5. "The journey of a thousand miles begins with a single Chair Pilates session."

6. "Embrace the simplicity of the chair; it's the tool that will elevate your Chair Pilates journey."

7. "Make your Chair Pilates tale one of commitment and development when you are still a beginning.

8. "Your journey in Chair Pilates is a canvas awaiting the brushstrokes of your effort and commitment."

9. "Don't compare your beginning to someone else's middle; every Chair Pilates journey is unique and inspiring."

10. "The key to success in your Chair Pilates practice is to start small.

11. "Every movement you make in the chair advances you toward your fitness objectives.

12. "As a beginner, you have the gift of limitless potential; your Chair Pilates practice is where that potential comes to life."

13. "In the realm of Chair Pilates, each beginner is a seeker of wellness and a champion of progress."

14. "The incredible Chair Pilates journey begins with the first step onto the chair.

15. "Your path with Chair Pilates is one of continuous development; challenges are stepping stones to growth.

16. "You build the foundation for a stronger and more exciting future with each gentle movement on the chair."

17. "Remember that every little effort is a victory worth celebrating in your Chair Pilates journey."

18. "Progress is not about perfection; it's about the persistence of a beginner willing to learn and grow."

19. "Every beginner's step you take should serve as evidence of your dedication to your Chair Pilates practice as an investment in your health.

20. "As a newbie, you are an inspiration; the light of your Chair Pilates journey illuminates the road to vitality."

May these quotes motivate and inspire you as you embark on your Chair Pilates journey as a beginner, reminding you that every small effort counts towards your progress and well-being.

READ THE MOTIVATIONAL QUOTES DAILY

CONCLUSION

As you turn the final pages of "Chair Pilates Strengthen Your Body, Transform Your Life," remember that your journey to enhanced well-being and vitality is an ongoing narrative of self-discovery and growth. This book has illuminated the path toward harnessing the power of the chair to nurture your body, mind, and spirit.

From humble beginnings as a beginner in Chair Pilates, you have embarked on a remarkable journey that has the potential to revolutionize your physical strength and inner balance. Every seated exercise you've embraced is a testament to your commitment to your own well-being.

Remember that progress is not defined solely by monumental leaps but by the consistency of small steps taken day by day. As you integrate Chair Pilates into your life, celebrate each movement as an investment in your health, a commitment to self-care, and a step toward realizing your full potential.

The chair that once seemed unassuming has become your trusted companion on this path of transformation. Its unwavering support has allowed you to explore new levels of strength, flexibility, and mindfulness. As you carry the lessons learned from these pages into your daily practice, let them serve as a reminder that your journey is unique and deeply personal.

The journey of Chair Pilates is more than physical; it's a dance of the body and spirit, a symphony of movement and mindfulness. With dedication and resilience, you have tapped into the wellspring of your own vitality, discovering that true strength emanates from within.

Your newfound awareness of your body, posture, and breath extends beyond the chair and enriches every facet of your life. Embrace this transformation with an open heart, for Chair Pilates has the power to touch every corner of your existence.

Thank you for allowing "Chair Pilates Strengthen Your Body, Transform Your Life" to be your guide on this transformative journey. May the lessons you've absorbed and the movements you've mastered continue to inspire you, reminding you that the chair is not just a piece of furniture, but a catalyst for personal growth and radiant well-being.

PILATES PROGRESS TRACKER

Daily Workout Progress Tracker

Pilates Goals •
For Seniors •
•

Exercise		How I felt today	Pilates Tracker
mon	4 3 3		◊◊◊◊ ◊◊◊◊
tue	4 3 4		◊◊◊◊ ◊◊◊◊
wed	4 3 3		◊◊◊◊ ◊◊◊◊
thu	4 3 3		◊◊◊◊ ◊◊◊◊
fri	4 3 3		◊◊◊◊ ◊◊◊◊
sat	4 3 3		◊◊◊◊ ◊◊◊◊
sun	4 3 3		◊◊◊◊ ◊◊◊◊

Daily Workout Progress Tracker

Pilates Goals •
For Seniors •
•

Exercise		How I felt today	Pilates Tracker
mon	4 _____ 3 _____ 3 _____	_____	◊◊◊◊ ◊◊◊◊
tue	4 _____ 3 _____ 4 _____	_____	◊◊◊◊ ◊◊◊◊
wed	4 _____ 3 _____ 3 _____	_____	◊◊◊◊ ◊◊◊◊
thu	4 _____ 3 _____ 3 _____	_____	◊◊◊◊ ◊◊◊◊
fri	4 _____ 3 _____ 3 _____	_____	◊◊◊◊ ◊◊◊◊
sat	4 _____ 3 _____ 3 _____	_____	◊◊◊◊ ◊◊◊◊
sun	4 _____ 3 _____ 3 _____	_____	◊◊◊◊ ◊◊◊◊

Daily Workout Progress Tracker

Pilates Goals •
For Seniors •
•

Exercise	How I felt today	Pilates Tracker

mon
4 ....
3 ....
3 ....

tue
4 ....
3 ....
4 ....

wed
4 ....
3 ....
3 ....

thu
4 ....
3 ....
3 ....

fri
4 ....
3 ....
3 ....

sat
4 ....
3 ....
3 ....

sun
4 ....
3 ....
3 ....

Daily Workout Progress Tracker

Pilates Goals •
For Seniors •
•

Exercise		How I felt today	Pilates Tracker
mon	4 ⸺ 3 ⸺ 3 ⸺	⸺ ⸺	◊◊◊◊ ◊◊◊◊
tue	4 ⸺ 3 ⸺ 4 ⸺	⸺ ⸺	◊◊◊◊ ◊◊◊◊
wed	4 ⸺ 3 ⸺ 3 ⸺	⸺ ⸺	◊◊◊◊ ◊◊◊◊
thu	4 ⸺ 3 ⸺ 3 ⸺	⸺ ⸺	◊◊◊◊ ◊◊◊◊
fri	4 ⸺ 3 ⸺ 3 ⸺	⸺ ⸺	◊◊◊◊ ◊◊◊◊
sat	4 ⸺ 3 ⸺ 3 ⸺	⸺ ⸺	◊◊◊◊ ◊◊◊◊
sun	4 ⸺ 3 ⸺ 3 ⸺	⸺ ⸺	◊◊◊◊ ◊◊◊◊

Daily Workout Progress Tracker

Pilates Goals •
For Seniors •
•

Exercise		How I felt today	Pilates Tracker
mon	4 .... 3 .... 3	....	◊◊◊◊ ◊◊◊◊
tue	4 .... 3 .... 4	....	◊◊◊◊ ◊◊◊◊
wed	4 .... 3 .... 3	....	◊◊◊◊ ◊◊◊◊
thu	4 .... 3 .... 3	....	◊◊◊◊ ◊◊◊◊
fri	4 .... 3 .... 3	....	◊◊◊◊ ◊◊◊◊
sat	4 .... 3 .... 3	....	◊◊◊◊ ◊◊◊◊
sun	4 .... 3 .... 3	....	◊◊◊◊ ◊◊◊◊

Daily Workout Progress Tracker

Pilates Goals •
For Seniors •
•

Exercise		How I felt today	Pilates Tracker
mon	4 3 3		◊◊◊◊ ◊◊◊◊
tue	4 3 4		◊◊◊◊ ◊◊◊◊
wed	4 3 3		◊◊◊◊ ◊◊◊◊
thu	4 3 3		◊◊◊◊ ◊◊◊◊
fri	4 3 3		◊◊◊◊ ◊◊◊◊
sat	4 3 3		◊◊◊◊ ◊◊◊◊
sun	4 3 3		◊◊◊◊ ◊◊◊◊

Daily Workout Progress Tracker

Pilates Goals •
For Seniors •
•

Exercise		How I felt today	Pilates Tracker
mon	4 _____ 3 _____ 3 _____	_____	◊◊◊◊ ◊◊◊◊
tue	4 _____ 3 _____ 4 _____	_____	◊◊◊◊ ◊◊◊◊
wed	4 _____ 3 _____ 3 _____	_____	◊◊◊◊ ◊◊◊◊
thu	4 _____ 3 _____ 3 _____	_____	◊◊◊◊ ◊◊◊◊
fri	4 _____ 3 _____ 3 _____	_____	◊◊◊◊ ◊◊◊◊
sat	4 _____ 3 _____ 3 _____	_____	◊◊◊◊ ◊◊◊◊
sun	4 _____ 3 _____ 3 _____	_____	◊◊◊◊ ◊◊◊◊

Daily Workout Progress Tracker

Pilates Goals •
For Seniors •
•

Exercise		How I felt today	Pilates Tracker
mon	4 _____ 3 _____ 3 _____	_____ _____ _____	◊◊◊◊ ◊◊◊◊
tue	4 _____ 3 _____ 4 _____	_____ _____ _____	◊◊◊◊ ◊◊◊◊
wed	4 _____ 3 _____ 3 _____	_____ _____ _____	◊◊◊◊ ◊◊◊◊
thu	4 _____ 3 _____ 3 _____	_____ _____ _____	◊◊◊◊ ◊◊◊◊
fri	4 _____ 3 _____ 3 _____	_____ _____ _____	◊◊◊◊ ◊◊◊◊
sat	4 _____ 3 _____ 3 _____	_____ _____ _____	◊◊◊◊ ◊◊◊◊
sun	4 _____ 3 _____ 3 _____	_____ _____ _____	◊◊◊◊ ◊◊◊◊

Daily Workout Progress Tracker

Pilates Goals •
For Seniors •
•

Exercise	How I felt today	Pilates Tracker
mon 4 / 3 / 3		◊◊◊◊ ◊◊◊◊
tue 4 / 3 / 4		◊◊◊◊ ◊◊◊◊
wed 4 / 3 / 3		◊◊◊◊ ◊◊◊◊
thu 4 / 3 / 3		◊◊◊◊ ◊◊◊◊
fri 4 / 3 / 3		◊◊◊◊ ◊◊◊◊
sat 4 / 3 / 3		◊◊◊◊ ◊◊◊◊
sun 4 / 3 / 3		◊◊◊◊ ◊◊◊◊

Daily Workout Progress Tracker

Pilates Goals •
For Seniors •
•

Exercise		How I felt today	Pilates Tracker
mon	4 _____ 3 _____ 3 _____	_____ _____ _____	◊◊◊◊ ◊◊◊◊
tue	4 _____ 3 _____ 4 _____	_____ _____ _____	◊◊◊◊ ◊◊◊◊
wed	4 _____ 3 _____ 3 _____	_____ _____ _____	◊◊◊◊ ◊◊◊◊
thu	4 _____ 3 _____ 3 _____	_____ _____ _____	◊◊◊◊ ◊◊◊◊
fri	4 _____ 3 _____ 3 _____	_____ _____ _____	◊◊◊◊ ◊◊◊◊
sat	4 _____ 3 _____ 3 _____	_____ _____ _____	◊◊◊◊ ◊◊◊◊
sun	4 _____ 3 _____ 3 _____	_____ _____ _____	◊◊◊◊ ◊◊◊◊

Daily Workout Progress Tracker

Pilates Goals •
For Seniors •
•

Exercise	How I felt today	Pilates Tracker
mon 4 ___ 3 ___ 3 ___		⬦⬦⬦⬦ ⬦⬦⬦⬦
tue 4 ___ 3 ___ 4 ___		⬦⬦⬦⬦ ⬦⬦⬦⬦
wed 4 ___ 3 ___ 3 ___		⬦⬦⬦⬦ ⬦⬦⬦⬦
thu 4 ___ 3 ___ 3 ___		⬦⬦⬦⬦ ⬦⬦⬦⬦
fri 4 ___ 3 ___ 3 ___		⬦⬦⬦⬦ ⬦⬦⬦⬦
sat 4 ___ 3 ___ 3 ___		⬦⬦⬦⬦ ⬦⬦⬦⬦
sun 4 ___ 3 ___ 3 ___		⬦⬦⬦⬦ ⬦⬦⬦⬦

Daily Workout Progress Tracker

Pilates Goals •
For Seniors •
•

Exercise		How I felt today	Pilates Tracker
mon	4 .... 3 .... 3	....	0000 0000
tue	4 .... 3 .... 4	....	0000 0000
wed	4 .... 3 .... 3	....	0000 0000
thu	4 .... 3 .... 3	....	0000 0000
fri	4 .... 3 .... 3	....	0000 0000
sat	4 .... 3 .... 3	....	0000 0000
sun	4 .... 3 .... 3	....	0000 0000

Daily Workout Progress Tracker

Pilates Goals •
For Seniors •
                •

Exercise	How I felt today	Pilates Tracker
mon 4 3 3		◊◊◊◊ ◊◊◊◊
tue 4 3 4		◊◊◊◊ ◊◊◊◊
wed 4 3 3		◊◊◊◊ ◊◊◊◊
thu 4 3 3		◊◊◊◊ ◊◊◊◊
fri 4 3 3		◊◊◊◊ ◊◊◊◊
sat 4 3 3		◊◊◊◊ ◊◊◊◊
sun 4 3 3		◊◊◊◊ ◊◊◊◊

Daily Workout Progress Tracker

Pilates Goals •
For Seniors •
•

Exercise		How I felt today	Pilates Tracker
mon	4 3 3		◊◊◊◊ ◊◊◊◊
tue	4 3 4		◊◊◊◊ ◊◊◊◊
wed	4 3 3		◊◊◊◊ ◊◊◊◊
thu	4 3 3		◊◊◊◊ ◊◊◊◊
fri	4 3 3		◊◊◊◊ ◊◊◊◊
sat	4 3 3		◊◊◊◊ ◊◊◊◊
sun	4 3 3		◊◊◊◊ ◊◊◊◊

Daily Workout Progress Tracker

Pilates Goals •
For Seniors •
•

Exercise		How I felt today	Pilates Tracker
mon	4 3 3		🌢🌢🌢🌢 🌢🌢🌢🌢
tue	4 3 4		🌢🌢🌢🌢 🌢🌢🌢🌢
wed	4 3 3		🌢🌢🌢🌢 🌢🌢🌢🌢
thu	4 3 3		🌢🌢🌢🌢 🌢🌢🌢🌢
fri	4 3 3		🌢🌢🌢🌢 🌢🌢🌢🌢
sat	4 3 3		🌢🌢🌢🌢 🌢🌢🌢🌢
sun	4 3 3		🌢🌢🌢🌢 🌢🌢🌢🌢

Daily Workout Progress Tracker

Pilates Goals •
For Seniors •
•

Exercise		How I felt today	Pilates Tracker
mon	4 _____ 3 _____ 3 _____		◊◊◊◊ ◊◊◊◊
tue	4 _____ 3 _____ 4 _____		◊◊◊◊ ◊◊◊◊
wed	4 _____ 3 _____ 3 _____		◊◊◊◊ ◊◊◊◊
thu	4 _____ 3 _____ 3 _____		◊◊◊◊ ◊◊◊◊
fri	4 _____ 3 _____ 3 _____		◊◊◊◊ ◊◊◊◊
sat	4 _____ 3 _____ 3 _____		◊◊◊◊ ◊◊◊◊
sun	4 _____ 3 _____ 3 _____		◊◊◊◊ ◊◊◊◊

Daily Workout Progress Tracker

Pilates Goals •
For Seniors •
 •

Exercise		How I felt today	Pilates Tracker
mon	4 .... 3 .... 3		◊◊◊◊ ◊◊◊◊
tue	4 .... 3 .... 4		◊◊◊◊ ◊◊◊◊
wed	4 .... 3 .... 3		◊◊◊◊ ◊◊◊◊
thu	4 .... 3 .... 3		◊◊◊◊ ◊◊◊◊
fri	4 .... 3 .... 3		◊◊◊◊ ◊◊◊◊
sat	4 .... 3 .... 3		◊◊◊◊ ◊◊◊◊
sun	4 .... 3 .... 3		◊◊◊◊ ◊◊◊◊

Daily Workout Progress Tracker

Pilates Goals •
For Seniors •
•

Exercise		How I felt today	Pilates Tracker
mon	4 3 3		○○○○ ○○○○
tue	4 3 4		○○○○ ○○○○
wed	4 3 3		○○○○ ○○○○
thu	4 3 3		○○○○ ○○○○
fri	4 3 3		○○○○ ○○○○
sat	4 3 3		○○○○ ○○○○
sun	4 3 3		○○○○ ○○○○

Daily Workout Progress Tracker

Pilates Goals   •
For Seniors   •
                   •

Exercise		How I felt today	Pilates Tracker
mon	4 3 3		◊◊◊◊ ◊◊◊◊
tue	4 3 4		◊◊◊◊ ◊◊◊◊
wed	4 3 3		◊◊◊◊ ◊◊◊◊
thu	4 3 3		◊◊◊◊ ◊◊◊◊
fri	4 3 3		◊◊◊◊ ◊◊◊◊
sat	4 3 3		◊◊◊◊ ◊◊◊◊
sun	4 3 3		◊◊◊◊ ◊◊◊◊

Daily Workout Progress Tracker

Pilates Goals •
For Seniors •
•

Exercise		How I felt today	Pilates Tracker
mon	4 .... 3 .... 3		◊◊◊◊ ◊◊◊◊
tue	4 .... 3 .... 4		◊◊◊◊ ◊◊◊◊
wed	4 .... 3 .... 3		◊◊◊◊ ◊◊◊◊
thu	4 .... 3 .... 3		◊◊◊◊ ◊◊◊◊
fri	4 .... 3 .... 3		◊◊◊◊ ◊◊◊◊
sat	4 .... 3 .... 3		◊◊◊◊ ◊◊◊◊
sun	4 .... 3 .... 3		◊◊◊◊ ◊◊◊◊

Daily Workout Progress Tracker

Pilates Goals •
For Seniors •
•

Exercise		How I felt today	Pilates Tracker
mon	4 / 3 / 3		◊◊◊◊ ◊◊◊◊
tue	4 / 3 / 4		◊◊◊◊ ◊◊◊◊
wed	4 / 3 / 3		◊◊◊◊ ◊◊◊◊
thu	4 / 3 / 3		◊◊◊◊ ◊◊◊◊
fri	4 / 3 / 3		◊◊◊◊ ◊◊◊◊
sat	4 / 3 / 3		◊◊◊◊ ◊◊◊◊
sun	4 / 3 / 3		◊◊◊◊ ◊◊◊◊

Daily Workout Progress Tracker

Pilates Goals •
For Seniors •
•

Exercise	How I felt today	Pilates Tracker
mon 4 3 3		◊◊◊◊ ◊◊◊◊
tue 4 3 4		◊◊◊◊ ◊◊◊◊
wed 4 3 3		◊◊◊◊ ◊◊◊◊
thu 4 3 3		◊◊◊◊ ◊◊◊◊
fri 4 3 3		◊◊◊◊ ◊◊◊◊
sat 4 3 3		◊◊◊◊ ◊◊◊◊
sun 4 3 3		◊◊◊◊ ◊◊◊◊

Daily Workout Progress Tracker

Pilates Goals •
For Seniors •
•

Exercise		How I felt today	Pilates Tracker
mon	4 3 3		◊◊◊◊ ◊◊◊◊
tue	4 3 4		◊◊◊◊ ◊◊◊◊
wed	4 3 3		◊◊◊◊ ◊◊◊◊
thu	4 3 3		◊◊◊◊ ◊◊◊◊
fri	4 3 3		◊◊◊◊ ◊◊◊◊
sat	4 3 3		◊◊◊◊ ◊◊◊◊
sun	4 3 3		◊◊◊◊ ◊◊◊◊

Daily Workout Progress Tracker

Pilates Goals	•
For Seniors	•
	•

Exercise		How I felt today	Pilates Tracker
mon	4 .... 3 .... 3		◊◊◊◊ ◊◊◊◊
tue	4 .... 3 .... 4		◊◊◊◊ ◊◊◊◊
wed	4 .... 3 .... 3		◊◊◊◊ ◊◊◊◊
thu	4 .... 3 .... 3		◊◊◊◊ ◊◊◊◊
fri	4 .... 3 .... 3		◊◊◊◊ ◊◊◊◊
sat	4 .... 3 .... 3		◊◊◊◊ ◊◊◊◊
sun	4 .... 3 .... 3		◊◊◊◊ ◊◊◊◊

Daily Workout Progress Tracker

Pilates Goals •
For Seniors •
•

Exercise	How I felt today	Pilates Tracker
mon 4 3 3		◊◊◊◊ ◊◊◊◊
tue 4 3 4		◊◊◊◊ ◊◊◊◊
wed 4 3 3		◊◊◊◊ ◊◊◊◊
thu 4 3 3		◊◊◊◊ ◊◊◊◊
fri 4 3 3		◊◊◊◊ ◊◊◊◊
sat 4 3 3		◊◊◊◊ ◊◊◊◊
sun 4 3 3		◊◊◊◊ ◊◊◊◊

Daily Workout Progress Tracker

Pilates Goals •
For Seniors •
•

Exercise		How I felt today	Pilates Tracker
mon	4 _____ 3 _____ 3 _____	_____	◊◊◊◊ ◊◊◊◊
tue	4 _____ 3 _____ 4 _____	_____	◊◊◊◊ ◊◊◊◊
wed	4 _____ 3 _____ 3 _____	_____	◊◊◊◊ ◊◊◊◊
thu	4 _____ 3 _____ 3 _____	_____	◊◊◊◊ ◊◊◊◊
fri	4 _____ 3 _____ 3 _____	_____	◊◊◊◊ ◊◊◊◊
sat	4 _____ 3 _____ 3 _____	_____	◊◊◊◊ ◊◊◊◊
sun	4 _____ 3 _____ 3 _____	_____	◊◊◊◊ ◊◊◊◊

Daily Workout Progress Tracker

Pilates Goals •
For Seniors •
•

Exercise	How I felt today	Pilates Tracker

mon
4 —
3 —
3 —

tue
4 —
3 —
4 —

wed
4 —
3 —
3 —

thu
4 —
3 —
3 —

fri
4 —
3 —
3 —

sat
4 —
3 —
3 —

sun
4 —
3 —
3 —

Daily Workout Progress Tracker

Pilates Goals •
For Seniors •
•

Exercise		How I felt today	Pilates Tracker
mon	4 .... 3 .... 3		◊◊◊◊ ◊◊◊◊
tue	4 .... 3 .... 4		◊◊◊◊ ◊◊◊◊
wed	4 .... 3 .... 3		◊◊◊◊ ◊◊◊◊
thu	4 .... 3 .... 3		◊◊◊◊ ◊◊◊◊
fri	4 .... 3 .... 3		◊◊◊◊ ◊◊◊◊
sat	4 .... 3 .... 3		◊◊◊◊ ◊◊◊◊
sun	4 .... 3 .... 3		◊◊◊◊ ◊◊◊◊

16176478R00028